Intermittent Fasting:

The Fundamental Guide To Sticking To Intermittent Fasting For Life.

author of this work can be in any fashion deemed liable for any hardship or damages that may befall them after undertaking information described herein.

Additionally, the information found on the following pages is intended for informational purposes only and should thus be considered, universal. As befitting its nature, the information presented is without assurance regarding its continued validity or interim quality. Trademarks that mentioned are done without written consent and can in no way be considered an endorsement from the trademark holder.

Table of Contents

Introduction 1

Does Intermittent Fasting really work?..............5

Benefits of Intermittent Fasting 11
It Removes Food/ Sugar Cravings 11
It Raises Insulin Sensitivity...12
It Is Very Simple Intermittent Fasting. 13
It is Flexible 14
Health Benefits 15
Rapid Weight Loss..16
Improves Brain Health 16
  Prevents Depression 16
  Increases Ketone Production 17
  Effective against Brain Trauma 17
  Prevents Huntington's Disease 17
  Detoxification 17

Intermittent Types and Fasting Schedules 19
16:8 Method 19
Eat-Stop-Eat 21
The Warrior Diet 23
Fat Loss Forever 24
Alternate Day Diet 25
Irregularly Skipping Meals 26

Specific Considerations When Implementing
Intermittent Fasting 29
Are there any indicators of someone whom intermittent fasting
may not be beneficial for? 32
Should a pregnant woman practice intermittent fasting?.........34
Should I fast if I am a diabetic? 34
Will intermittent fasting affect my menstrual cycle and fertility?
....35

The Do's And Don'ts 37

How does intermittent fasting work? 38

Do's and don'ts of intermittent fasting for women 39

Do keep tabs on your hormone health. 39

Don't diet. 40

Do focus on fats. 40

Don't workout intensely. 41

Don't make fat loss your main goal. 42

Do start slow. 43

Don't continue if you feel bad. 43

Do enlist the support of a professional. 43

The Biggest Mistakes to Avoid 45

Continuing to Eat Crap Food 45

Not Keeping Yourself Busy 45

You Set Goals Too High 46

You Fear Going Hungry 46

You Spend Your Days Staring at the Clock 46

Obsessing Over the Sum of the Parts 47

Common Myths of Intermittent Fasting 49

Fasting is Basically Starving Yourself 50

Fasting Will Slow Down Your Metabolism 50

You Will Gain Back The Weight You Lost After Eating 51

Fasting Only Helps You Lose Water Weight 52

Having Less Energy When Fasting 52

Fat Makes You Fat 52

Your Brain Will Stop Functioning Without Carbs 53

You Need Supplements To Make Up for Lack of Food 53

Fasting and Training Are a Bad Combination 54

When Fasting Is Not For Everyone 54

You should not try intermittent fasting if: 54

Conclusion 57

Introduction

You probably want to give intermittent fasting a try. At the very least, it provides a default choice in the face of any confusion about whether what you are eating is counterproductive or not: "When in doubt, don't eat." Here's how to get started:

Map out a day where you can go at least about 14 hours without solid food (water, tea, and black coffee are okay). This usually involves the period after you've finished dinner and then throughout the night. But you can use whatever setup is easiest to implement, given your life schedule. The actual time blocks depend on your personal work and sleep routine, of course.

The fast cannot usually involve any calories (unless you're doing a partial fast); this would disrupt the fasting metabolism (in which your blood-sugar or glucose levels are maintained without the input of food. Tea or coffee without cream or sugar is generally okay, but a purist might insist on no caffeine, which exerts a powerful effect on the central nervous system (thus, you could argue, changing the hormonal milieu for the fast). Most of us have to work or have responsibilities during most fasts, so a little coffee or green tea during the intermittent fast is a reasonable compromise and poses no harm.

Upon awakening, in the usual fasted evening scenario, you skip breakfast and, if so inclined, start the day only with a cup of joe or tea. As we mentioned, a lump of sugar and big splash of cream in the coffee will tend to send the food signal to the body, in part by raising insulin levels, so that's generally considered a "cheat," or you might consider this a partial or moderate fast.

The USDA Nutrient Database does indicate that tea and even black coffee are not 100 percent calorie-free (two calories per eight ounces, in fact). An intermittent fasting purist may insist on only water or reliably calorie-free drinks during the fast, but we might be splitting hairs a bit too finely here. You'll still be getting some of the metabolic benefits of fasting by restricting calories a lot.

The science also supports a fasted workout. Therefore, the next step would be to hit the gym hungry for your favorite high-intensity weight regimen. To many beginner and veteran athletes, this might seem counterintuitive, even scary, but it actually feels good and the athlete tends to adapt to lifting weights on just sleep, water, and coffee (in my case). What is the science?

For one, a 2010 study in the Journal of Physiology took three groups of young men and fed them a high-fat, high-calorie diet for more than a month.

They divided them into three groups: one group fasted and trained (four times a week cycling); another group trained on carbohydrate fuels, like a high-carb breakfast followed by energy drinks during exercise; and the third (control) group did nothing.

The control group gained about seven pounds in six weeks, predictably. The carb-fed group gained about three pounds, but the athletes training in the fasted state didn't gain any weight, even when they were pigging out around the training and fasting.

Among the fasters, several biomarkers improved at a higher rate than in the carb group, including insulin sensitivity and the muscle adaptations for quickly turning over the increased fatty acids in the diet.

You can also do endurance training in the fasted state. This appears on the face of it, and from my experience as a former endurance athlete when I usually stuffed food like gels or bananas in my pocket, to be much harder to do when fasting than short-term high-intensity weight training. After 80 minutes of, say, hard riding, you could bonk, and there are good physiological reasons for that, such as because all the glycogen—your internal storage depot of starch in the muscles and liver—has been depleted by the fasting and exercise itself. It does depend on the intensity level of the exercise, and how well you have previously adapted to fasting. You could also save this kind of training for the no fasting days, unless you're very adapted to it.

Or, you don't have to train; you'll still enjoy some of the benefits of intermittent fasting.

In addition, growing scientific evidence points to the outstanding benefits of this diet for human health and longevity. Based on evolutionary biology, we now know that the human body evolved to thrive on specific foods and a certain feeding cycle. The premise of the fastening diet is to revive these primal dietary features and provide guidance on how to apply them in your diet.

Does Intermittent Fasting really work?

Intermittent fasting is intended on allowing your body to be hungry enough to consume from stored energy without being in starvation. Starvation mode is when your body has lacked calories for so long that when you do eat instead of using the energy the body will immediately store it in reserves just in case another starvation happens. This is why the fad of "yo-yo dieting" was so unsuccessful – people put themselves into starvation and would actually gain weight once they began eating again. This is also why it is important to have a proper fasting schedule since you want to avoid starvation mode.

Research into weight loss has been around since the 1920's. Studies involving fasting have shown the same results with everything from fruit flies to monkeys. Fasting actually affects what you lose. Most diets will cause you to lose fat, water and even a little muscle but intermittent fasting has been shown to actually concentrate your weight loss on fat alone. It does this by choosing where the best energy source is during your fasted state. Normally your body would choose glucose in the bloodstream or temporarily stored glycogen in the liver since they are easier to process.

When you fast these become unavailable which forces the body to choose the only other stored energy available – fat. This is especially true with working out. If you have tried to drink protein shakes before a workout and have not noticed any improvement this is because your body is choosing to consume the shake rather than any excess body fat you have. Working out in a fasted state forces the body to consume fat to keep up your energy levels.

When you fast, in addition to making your body burn fat you also increase your sensitivity to insulin. When we think of insulin most people think of it as something diabetics need, the reason they need it is because either their body has become desensitized to their own or they are not producing enough. Insulin regulates the amount of glucose in the blood and those who are overweight often find their levels are not right because the body produces so much that it becomes desensitized. By fasting we can increase the sensitivity since your body is being deprived of the readily available glucose it would have from eating too often.

This is a very important tool since with desensitization your body may choose to store more of the glycogen it's making rather than burning it causing your blood glucose level to fluctuate in ways it shouldn't. As the problem of obesity grows worldwide the amount of research into dietary phenomenon grows also. Fasting has its own plethora of science behind why it really does work. So what happens on a day where you don't fast?

The regular intake of food allows the body to keep using the glucose in the bloodstream as it is energy source. Insulin sensitivity will be at normal (or in some cases desensitized) levels. Easily processable glycogen stores will be full which means any additional energy the body receives will go into storage as fat. It won't matter if you eat 20 calories or 200 over your needed amount, anything excess becomes fat and your body has no need to consume any stored energy.

Fasting can be seen as a training method, you are training your body to be more efficient in how it consumes the nutrition you give it. The physiological reasons alone are good enough, but what about the benefits that also come from losing weight? Those who weigh less enjoy a much lower risk for a variety of different health issues, they're also seen as socially superior (something controversial but unfortunately true) and the emotional benefits of having lost excess weight can also lead to an overall happier life. Weight loss can also lead to improvement in other areas – heavier people find they have bad knees or back issues from the strain of carrying extra weight.

The advantages of fasting which might be stated earlier are just the typical ones. The fact in this is a part of the benefits that are mentioned above is always that each individual who have advantages from fasting a result of the belief that everyone is exclusive. And absolutely, each individual who will about to fast will get the matter that he/she desires to be!

Intermittent fasting has grown to be quite the sensation right now. You can find were recent reports that showed that with somebody that has tried it, they dropped a few pounds, and increased how much their own health. Simply to present you with a perception, intermittent fasting is a style of eating where you stand likely to alternative your intervals of fasting, oftentimes only having water as well as on the opposite hand, non-fasting is simply eating precisely what you choose no matter how fatty food is.

Quite simply, a person can eat all sorts of things he wants throughout a 24-hour period and fast for the following 24 hours. This technique to weight control is based on the research along with the ethical practices across the world. When the person will going to present an intermittent fasting he then will certainly get what he could be wanting.

You are likely to notice that there are numerous kinds of intermittent fasts. You can find that we now have 2 kinds of intermittent fasting these are the commonly used as well as the easiest. First could be the daily fasting in which the person only grows to take in once just about every 20-28 hours within a 4-hour period. The second reason is fasting for 1-3x every week, also referred to as different day fasting, when a man or woman eats anything he desires on a single day along with fast the entire of the following day.

Intermittent fasting has many beneficial effects as tried on wildlife like animals and also primates. A report finds out that a man who does the fasting will about to decrease the levels of insulin that he's having and will about to improve the resistance of the

8

neurons inside the brain. In 2008, a survey was developed about intermittent fasting plus it established that the lifespan of an individual improves of 40.4% and 56.6% in C. The public that does the various day fasting has indicated that they tend to give up more weight as opposed to ones who are getting the normal diet. Along with the 2009 study showed that intermittent fasting around the rats improved the rats' survival after having a continual heart failure via pro-angiogenic and then these people have a lengthy lifespan also.

The study only caution is usually that there are few studies which have been completed to the people who do intermittent fasts. The results with the upper frequency within the composition of the body and workouts are interesting and not yet explored in your community of research. However, there are many positive results. Very last month, a study that had been made by the National Academy of Sciences posted a book that ensures that reducing calories 30% per day will planning to increase the memory perform from the old people. In the past year 2007, the journal Free Radical Biology & Medicine indicates to the public the fact that those who are having to deal with bronchial asthma who quicker had much fewer symptoms and in addition they reduction in the markers in the blood that they're having in comparison to the first.

Benefits of Intermittent Fasting

As they were some benefits of the fasting, there are people who are utilizing this to lose excess weight plus some are using it to raise their health problems. Some individuals also say that fasting is a strategy to look young and possess a longer life. This is why that this procedure sounds intriguing to my opinion. The simple fact is that same reasons why I would like to reveal the intermittent fasting benefits together with you.

Really, this ingesting style isn't that challenging. Accusation in court is essentially eating whatever you need within a day and then the overnight you are likely to fast. It indicates no food! (Besides water).It is very completely different from our usual eating habits. However, you can see it as being an extreme weight-loss but fasting is really a great means for anyone to search and feel great inside and outside!

Periodic fasting can help clear up the mind and strengthen the body and the spirit. Although people commonly believe that depriving yourself of food for too long is unhealthy for you, scientists have proven that Intermittent Fasting provides many benefits.

It Removes Food/ Sugar Cravings

A lot of the time when we feel "hungry" we actual feel cravings for sugars and carbohydrates. When you are fasting, your body will switch from using carbohydrates as fuel to using your burned fat stores instead. Your body will learn that carbohydrates aren't needed for energy and that it can use the fat already stored in your body for energy.

Aside from removing your sugar cravings, you will also remove the cravings for the food itself. Because your body "will realize" that it doesn't need food for energy, it won't crave it too often. Thus, by removing all the hunger triggers you'll get through the day. This is why the myth of "eating 5-6 times a day" is not true. When you eat 5-6 times a day and even implement carbohydrates, you'll never allow your body to burn fat. This is due the fact that the body will use the carbohydrates as energy first before using the fat in your body.

It Raises Insulin Sensitivity

Insulin is a hormone in the body that regulates the function of cells. Insulin is made by the pancreas and is secreted when we eat food. It then binds to signal cells and allows our body to store the sugars as energy. The less insulin we need to store these sugars, the more sensitive we become to insulin, and the better insulin can do its work in the long term.

When we eat 5 to 6 times a day, our insulin levels stay too high for a long period of time. This insulin won't be used effectively, and this will eventually raise our resistance to it. When we are resistant to insulin, we can develop type 2 diabetes or prediabetes. Diabetes is a disease that prevents us from storing all the sugars we consume, because the insulin that our pancreas produces won't work properly. When this happens the sugars will not be stored as energy and will remain in our bloodstream, leading to high blood sugar levels and hardening of the blood vessels.

This can eventually cause kidney diseases, heart attacks, erectile dysfunction, and loss of vision, strokes, nerve damage and much more critical health problems. However, when you fast for a long period of time, you are forcing your body to use the fat stored as energy and not the food that you are digesting. This will allow your body to create less insulin and therefore become more insulin sensitive, preventing all these problems.

It Is Very Simple Intermittent Fasting.

It doesn't require much effort to plan the quantity, quality and timing of your meals. Any active gym practitioners put much effort in preparing their meals to track their calories. This method is fine by itself, but can be very energy draining and time consuming.

In this day and age, we don't have much time anymore due to our fast-paced, demanding lifestyles, so it is better to save time by eliminating unnecessary duties like meal prepping. When you are fasting you only need to worry about 1 or 2 meals, and you always know at which times of the day you are going to eat. This will allow you to spend a greater amount of time on more important tasks.

When you realize that meal prepping is not so important, you will notice that you are still getting the same results with less effort. This is also called the 80/20 principle. 80% of our results come from 20% of our efforts. It is up to us to find out which 20% matters. And often, meal prepping doesn't belong to the 20%.

Also, because you are eating one or two large meals a say, it won't be necessary to constantly keep track of your calories. And it is much more difficult to over consume your daily calories in one or two meals (unless you are eating junk food of course).

Note: If you are a professional bodybuilder, then this doesn't apply to you. You can't expect to enter competitions and win them while not staying as lean as possible. So, for those people who are entering competitions, I highly recommend that you keep track of all your calories and stick to what works!

It is Flexible

Having strict meal plans can be very difficult to sustain. Most of us have important and demanding jobs that don't allow us to eat when we need to. Rather, we get breaks at the moments that we don't really need them. Or we are traveling a lot, which keeps us from eating our meals when we need to. Fasting, however, provides a huge amount of flexibility. Because you have a short time window, you can choose when to eat. This will give you the opportunity to eat when it suits you best.

For me personally, it becomes really hard to plan my meals and stay on track of my meal schedule when I am traveling or working. Fasting allows me to go without eating for a long time and simply eat when it suits me best.

Health Benefits

Studies show that Intermittent Fasting has many health benefits. Individuals who are overweight or suffer from diseases like diabetes may benefit the most from Intermittent Fasting.

Overweight people or individuals with type 2 diabetes will lose more weight and improve their heart health when they fast occasionally. Even if they don't reduce calorie in- take (but rather stay in maintenance mode), they will see results. But of course, if you want to maximize your results, make sure you're in a small calorie deficit and eat healthy foods.

Other health benefits are:
- Limiting inflammation
- Reducing blood pressure
- Improve pancreatic function
- Protects against cardiovascular disease
- Reduce total cholesterol and LDL levels
- Improves insulin sensitivity

While Intermittent Fasting itself is healthy for diabetic people, it can be harmful due to the fact that you are depriving yourself of nutrients at certain times of the day. So again, Intermittent Fasting is healthy for you if you are diabetic, but be sure to consult your doctor first!

Rapid Weight Loss

As stated earlier, normally you'll receive energy from the carbohydrates that you consume. This will prevent you from burning the fat you have stored in your body. Yet when you are fasting, you are forcing your body to use the fat you have stored for energy. This by itself will lead to instant and rapid fat loss, which means that you will not only look better, but actually be healthier too.

Also, because you are fasting for 1 or 2 days every week, you are automatically cutting many calories (1000-4500 calories a week). This will result in massive and rapid weight loss, allowing you to lose approximately 0.5-1 pound a week! You will be able to keep your muscle and lose the fat, resulting in amazing body transformations.

Improves Brain Health

Intermittent Fasting also has many benefits for the brain. It improves your memory functioning and accelerates learning. It also boosts your BDNF (Brain Derived Neurotropic Factor), which in turn builds your brain tissues. This will make you smarter and help you gain stronger muscles.

Some other benefits are:

Prevents Depression

Researchers have shown that having low BDNF is linked to depression. Good against Alzheimer's Disease Research was conducted with 2 mice with Alzheimer's disease. One was Intermittent Fasting and the other mouse followed the standard diet (both were consuming the same amount of calories).

They were put in a Morris water maze, and the mouse who was Intermittent Fasting found his way much faster than the other.

Increases Ketone Production

Intermittent Fasting actively stimulates the production of ketones. Ketones are acids that are made by the body to help it use fat as an energy source instead of using carbohydrates as an energy source.

Effective against Brain Trauma

Fasting reduces the mitochondrial dysfunction, oxidative stress and cognitive decline that usually result from brain traumas.

Prevents Huntington's Disease

This disease will deplete your BDNF levels, but research showed that fasting rats with Huntington's disease kept their BDNF levels stable.

Detoxification

It is intended to cleanse the human system of toxins that accumulated during rapid fast-food and heavy meals.

Intermittent Types and Fasting Schedules

While the core ideas behind the various forms of intermittent fasting are all the same, there are quite a few different ways to go about it. Your best bet is to try a few and see which one your body naturally responds to the easiest.

16:8 Method

This method involves fasting for 16 hours for men, or 14 hours for women, before allowing a reasonable number of calories for the remaining 8 to 10 hours. During this period, you should only consume items that have zero calories including black coffee (a splash of cream is fine), water, diet soda, and sugar-free gum. The easiest way to attempt this schedule is to stop eating after dinner in the evening and wait 14 or 16 hours from there. This means skipping breakfast and picking things up in the early afternoon.

Again, the specifics of when you fast are not nearly as important as ensuring that you fast for the same period of time as regularly as possible. If you vary your fasting period too much, it can lead to an erratic change in your hormones, which among other things; make it much more difficult for your body to shed any excess weight. If you find yourself without the time required to eat a proper meal to break the fast normally, ensure you at least eat something to keep your body on the correct cycle.

If you are exercising, as well as intermittently fasting, it is important to ensure that you are eating more carbohydrates than fats while you are working out, while on days you are not exercising the opposite is true. It is important to ensure that every day you keep your protein intake at a steady level. Stay away from processed foods whenever possible.

One of the biggest benefits of this type of fasting is that it's extremely flexible so that it will work for a wide variety schedules. Most people find it helpful to either eat two large meals during the 8 or 10-hour period feeding period or split that time into three smaller meals as that is the way most people are already programmed.

On days you are exercising as well as fasting, it is important to try and always break your fast with a mix of protein, vegetables, and fruit. If you generally go to the gym directly after you have broken your fast, it is important to include enough carbohydrates to give your muscles the energy they need to get the most out of your workout.

If you are planning to exercise, it is usually best to start the early afternoon healthy with a medium calorie meal. Then, exercise within three hours before eating a larger meal soon afterward. In this larger meal, it is important to add a larger portion of complex carbohydrates. You can even have a little dessert as long as it is in moderation. Remember, fasting is different than dieting.

On days you do not plan on exercising, it is important to adjust your caloric intake appropriately. Start by limiting your carbohydrate intake, and instead focus on eating lots of protein, dark green, leafy vegetables and fruit in moderation. Unlike on days you are exercising, the first meal you eat on rest days should be your largest regarding caloric intake with this one meal counting for about 40 percent of your daily total.

Remember, during this meal, you should be taking in more protein than anything else. For your final meal during rest days, it is important to include a protein source that will take lots of time to digest which in turn means it will keep you full for more of your fast the following morning. It also provides the body with enough stored amino acids to prevent it from breaking down muscle during the fast.

Eat-Stop-Eat

This form of fasting can be considered the most beneficial to those who are already eating healthy but want to give their weight loss an extra boost. On this type of program, you don't eat anything one or two days a week. During this period, you should only consume things that have zero calories including black coffee (a splash of cream is fine), water, diet soda, and sugar-free gum.

When you are finished fasting, it is important not to eat too much more than normal and always to avoid binging as extended periods of fast/binge cycles can cause serious damage to your body. As always, it is important to practice moderation and self-control to get the most out of the fasting cycle.

This fast cycle works on the assumption that in to lose a pound of weight a week, all you need to do is give up 3,500 calories. So, it might be best to get it out of the way in two quick bursts rather than fasting for a portion of every single day. This fasting plan emphasizes resistance weight training for maximum benefits.

Going a full day without eating can be difficult for some people at first, but it is perfectly acceptable to work up to a full day of fasting by holding out as long as possible and increasing that amount of time with practice. A good way to start is by choosing days that you know don't have any prior food commitments. Beginning a fasting program on a day when you know you have a lunch meeting is just a bad idea.

When first starting this fast cycle, fatigue, headaches or feelings of anger or anxiousness are all common side-effects and should be considered a good stopping point for your current fast. These side-effects will diminish as your body adjusts to the new cycle.

After going a full day without any calories, it will be natural to have the desire to binge during your fist meal. You must have the self-control to fight these urges since not only is binging bad for you; it can easily undo all your hard work from the previous 24 hours. Practice self-discipline and make your fasting worth the effort.

The Warrior Diet

The Warrior Diet takes the 16:8 Program and kicks it up a notch by recommending that you fast for roughly 20 hours out of each day followed by one meal where you get all your calories in the four remaining hours of the day.

This form of intermittent fasting follows the belief that humans are naturally nocturnal eaters. Therefore, eating at night helps the body more easily process the nutrients it needs. In this case, fasting is a bit of a misnomer as during the 20-hour period you are allowed to eat a serving of raw vegetables or fruits and maybe a serving of protein if you just can't otherwise continue.

This works because it causes the body's natural sympathetic nervous system to activate a flight or fight response which in turns increases your natural levels of alertness, and increases energy while at the same time increasing the amount of fat burned. The large meal each evening then allows the body to focus on repairing itself and improving its muscles. When following the Warrior Diet, it is important to start each evening meal with vegetables, followed by protein, fat, and carbohydrates.

This form of fasting is popular for two reasons. First, the fact that a few small and reasonable snacks are allowed during the fasting process making this type of fasting attractive to those who are attempting the practice for the first time. Second, nearly everyone who attempts this form of fasting reports a significant amount of increased energy throughout the day as well as increase in the amount of fat lost per week.

On the other hand, the relatively strict nature of this diet can make it difficult for some people to follow for long periods of time. The timing of the large meal can also make it difficult for some people to follow because it can naturally interfere with some social engagements. Finally, some people don't like having to eat their food in a specific order. Try it for yourself and see what works for you.

Fat Loss Forever

This form of intermittent fasting combines elements of several other styles of fasting to create something rather unique. The good news is that you get a cheat day every week. The bad news is that it is followed by a one and a half day fast with the remainder of the week being split between 16:8 and 20:4 fasting.

For this diet, it is important to schedule your exercise rest days for the second part of the 36-hour cycle. Otherwise, it is important to stay as busy on these days as possible to help combat your hunger. If you find it hard to control your appetite on cheat days, then this form of intermittent fasting may not be for you since it requires you to go from sixty to zero quickly and regularly.

Also, it is important not to try and last 36 hours without eating food all at once. You will need to build up your body's tolerance for fasting. As such, it is usually better to start with another form of intermittent fasting and work up to the Fat Loss Forever method after your body has already gotten out of the habit of eating every three or four hours.

Remember to always fast responsibly, and never push your body to the point where you feel physically ill. Also, remember it is important to fast on a routine to allow your body the time it needs to adjust to the change.

Alternate Day Diet

This form of intermittent fasting actually means you never have to go long without food, if you so choose. Every other day you eat normally, and on the off-days, you simply consume one-fifth of the calories you consume on the normal days. The average daily caloric consumption is between 2,000 and 2,500 calories which mean that the average off-day varies between 400 and 500 calories. If you enjoy exercising every day, then this form of intermittent fasting may not be for you since you will have to severely limit your workouts on off-days.

When you first start this form of intermittent fasting, the easiest way to make it through the low-calorie days is by trying any one of a variety of protein shakes. It is important to work back to 'real' natural foods on these days because they will always be healthier than the shakes.

This form of intermittent fasting is all about losing weight. Those who try it tend to average between two and three pounds lost per week. If you attempt the Alternate Day Diet, it is extremely important to eat regularly on your full-calorie days. Binging will not only negate any progress you have made, but it can also cause serious damage to your body if continued over time.

Irregularly Skipping Meals

If you are interested in trying out the benefits of intermittent fasting for yourself, but you have an irregular schedule or are not sure if it is for you, then skipping a meal or two now and then may be the type of intermittent fasting for you. As previously discussed, getting into a fasting routine is important to see the maximum results for your effort, but that doesn't mean occasionally fasting doesn't come with some benefits as well.

What's more, once you have tried skipping a meal now and then you can see for yourself just how easy it is which in turn can lead to more positive changes down the line. With so many intermittent fasting options available the odds are good that one fits your schedule, so give it a try. What have you got to lose (besides a few pounds)?

Specific Considerations When Implementing Intermittent Fasting

You've now got a thorough understanding of the background of intermittent fasting, the scientifically based evidence of its benefits, how to do it, and how to work this cycle of eating into your life.

There are some considerations as to who may or may not benefit from intermittent fasting. There are a lot of women (and men) who have gotten great weight loss results using some form of fasting and cycled eating. However, just like any diet and exercise program or regimen, intermittent fasting is not for everyone, and it's important you practice the proper weight loss plan for your body and your specific goals. Intermittent fasting is certainly not something that everyone needs to do, but it's a helpful tool in the weight loss battle that so many women struggle with. It can be easily implemented in many women's daily lives and used to promote greater overall health and well-being, but it can, in some cases, be misused as well.

There are a few pre-requisites that if followed, will make your intermittent fasting weight loss journey easier and more successful, and make you a good candidate for reaping the most benefits from this program. These include the following:

•Get enough sleep on a regular basis.

•Minimize stress in your daily life.

•Make sure lifestyle activity is within a normal range—not too much or too little daily movement and/or exercise.

•Be fat adapted. This means that your body can easily access and burn stored fat throughout the day when it's needed to provide energy.

So, how can you tell if you're already considered fat adapted? No blood test can give you this answer, but there are a few simple questions you can ask yourself that should be able to provide you with an indication of your level of fat adaptability:

•Can you go 3 hours or more without eating? Would skipping a meal be an incredibly difficult physical and mental struggle for you?

•On a normal day, do you feel your energy level stays consistent throughout the day? Do you need to take an afternoon nap or is it just something you enjoy doing now and again?

•Are you able to perform fairly vigorous physical activity like steady walking, jogging, or light exercise without first consuming carbohydrates for energy?

•Do you frequently suffer from headaches, mental exhaustion, and mental fog?

Someone whose body is fat adapted can usually skip meals with little effort on their part. They have consistent energy and do not require an afternoon nap to make it through the second portion of their day. They are able to be moderately active and perform physical activities like brisk walking, jogging, hiking, biking, and swimming without needing to fuel their body beforehand with carbohydrates, and they do not suffer from the mental fog, headaches, and exhaustion that a person whose body is more sugar dependent may.

Some of you are lucky and are genetically predisposed to be a fat burning machine! Others of you may not be, and your genetics may require more effort than the first group to reach this state of fat burning and freedom from sugar and carbohydrate dependence. Luckily for all of us, your genes are not final! They don't define you, and they can be altered! Through your behavior and your lifestyle choices, you have the ability to turn on and off various genes in your genetic code that can lead to the physical results you desire. There are numerous versions of the future person you may become, and it's always up to you to make the decisions that will ultimately lead to who you will become. You are responsible for making choices and living a lifestyle that will promote and direct your genes toward fat loss, building muscle, and overall wellness. Following an intermittent fasting style of eating will put you on the path to achieving this longevity of life and general wellness of the body.

If you feel that you may be lacking in the fat-adaptability department and want to give yourself the best start to your intermittent fasting protocol, it can benefit you to try eating the paleo style diet for 3 weeks before beginning your cycles of fasting and eating. This basically means you'll eliminate sugar, grains, legumes, and vegetable oils from your diet for 3 weeks prior to beginning intermittent fasting. This should be the push your body needs to become more efficient in drawing upon fat stores for energy rather than relying on dietary sugar for fuel. Again, this step is not necessary for your pursuit of weight loss through intermittent fasting, but it can set you up for the most success in the shortest amount of time.

Are there any indicators of someone whom intermittent fasting may not be beneficial for?

Intermittent fasting may not be a great protocol to follow for someone who is susceptible to eating disorders. If you've had a problem with disordered eating at any point in your life, it might be beneficial for you to explore multiple weight loss plans before deciding what works best for you. If intermittent fasting seems like the best choice for your lifestyle, do take the time to pay special attention to the amount of food you're consuming when you are not in your fasting periods, just to be sure you do not continuously deny yourself nutrition.

Intermittent fasting is considered a stressor on your body systems. You're using planned fasting and hunger to ignite metabolic processes within your body that respond to these stressors. For this reason, someone with a multitude of other stressors may not fare as well while following an intermittent fasting protocol. Mental stress, physical stress, and emotional stress can all hinder your mental ability to properly complete your fasting cycles as well as your body's physical ability to lose weight. Adding this new stressor can compound any other existing stressors, which won't be the most effective way to begin your weight loss journey.

Intermittent fasting may not be beneficial for someone with a cortisol regulation disorder. If you're actively monitoring your cortisol levels with your doctor or if you think you may have an issue with cortisol regulation it would be best to seek a professional opinion before implementing a fast into your weight loss regimen. Fasting raises cortisol levels in the body, and in a healthy individual, this poses no threat or health issue. Someone with a cortisol dysregulation can have serious side effects if their levels become excessive, and an activity that boosts production of cortisol may not be right for these people. If you think you may have an issue with cortisol regulation, visit your doctor before starting a program and find out for sure. You may have an issue with cortisol regulation if you retain excess belly fat, consistently lack enough sleep, persistently suffer from low-grade stress, and rely on caffeine to keep you awake and energized each day.

Should a pregnant woman practice intermittent fasting?

There haven't been many studies done on the effects of fasting on pregnant women on their growing fetus. One study17 that followed pregnant women fasting for Ramadan showed that these women had a decrease in the development and growth of their placentas, but the slower growth was more efficient. The developing fetus grew as normal, but the women had much smaller reserves of nutrients in their bodies. Although this (and a few other) studies show that short-term fasting is probably safe during pregnancy, it is most likely a better idea to wait until after giving birth. Fasting during pregnancy is not necessary (except in these cases of religiously required fasts) and is probably not beneficial to the woman or her growing baby.

Should I fast if I am a diabetic?

This is a gray area and should be reviewed with your doctor before you begin. Women have a more difficult time regulating their blood sugar than men and can be more severely affected by a drop in blood sugar. There have been accounts of men who were classified as diabetic using intermittent fasting to control their blood sugar levels, lose weight, and effectively beat type-2 diabetes, but there have been no such accounts for women.

Will intermittent fasting affect my menstrual cycle and fertility?

Humans are highly biologically effective at adapting to their environments. When proper nutrition is not available, it is more work for a woman's body to create new life and provide nutrition for the baby once it's born. For this reason, women are biologically designed to respond to the presence or scarcity of available food by altering some aspects of fertility. There haven't been clinical studies directly comparing the effects of intermittent fasting on female fertility. These studies do have to look at, mostly, and compare fertility changes due to extreme fasting circumstances like famine or anorexia—which are not truly comparable to planned and purposeful intermittent fasting. These studies do show a link between decreased fertility, the loss of a menstrual cycle, and fasting, but the differences between these scenarios and intermittent fasting should be considered. There is currently too little evidence-based clinical information on the relationship between intermittent fasting and female reproductive health to definitively say if it is beneficial, neutral, or harmful.

The Do's And Don'ts

Over the last several years, there has been a lot of buzz around the concept of intermittent fasting (IF) and for good reason. Many people swear by intermittent fasting to decrease body fat, increase energy and focus, assist in detoxification, keep aging at bay, and even protect them against chronic disease. In fact, there is evidence to suggest that intermittent fasting can decrease the risk of certain diseases such as type 2 diabetes, cardiovascular disease, and even cancer.

In general, intermittent fasting is a way to manipulate the timing of your food intake to allow for periods of time spent in a fasting state which requires the body to turn to a different source of fuel – body fat. Not only that, but during times of fasting, blood glucose is lowered, growth hormone is triggered, hunger regulating hormones like leptin and ghrelin are normalized, detoxification becomes a focus, and the digestive system gets a rest and reset too. While our current society may find going large amounts of time without food to be against what we know, various cultures throughout history practice fasting regularly because of its amazing mind, body, and health benefits, not to mention our ancestors in the paleolithic area no doubt went through regular feasts and famines while hunting for food.

How does intermittent fasting work?

There are a few different methods of IF, all of which are effective, so it's more a matter of individual preference as to how someone incorporates it into their life.

Some examples include:

Scheduling one day per week to fast for 24 hours. The other 6 days have a normal food intake.

Schedule alternating days to eat very little (500-600 calories) and the other days have a normal food intake.

Scheduling a daily fast of 14-18 hours. This can be done by skipping breakfast or just condensing all 3 meals into an 6-10 hour window.

Do's and don'ts of intermittent fasting for women

Do keep tabs on your hormone health.

The biggest risk women have with intermittent fasting is with their hormones. Women hormones play a very delicate balancing act on a repeated 28-day cycle (on average). Sometimes the slightest change in our diet, health, mindset, environment, toxin exposure, or stress-level can cause hormonal imbalance to occur leading to further health issues down the road. If not done properly, intermittent fasting could easily become one of these triggers for hormonal imbalance because of the stress it can cause on your body.

It's not only the sex hormones that can be affected. Cortisol and thyroid hormones are also very important to monitor, especially if you have had past issues with thyroid disorders or adrenal fatigue.

Following the steps listed below will help tremendously in keeping your hormones balanced and stress level regulated. It is also very important to check on the state of your hormones before you even begin. If you are already dealing with a hormonal imbalance of any kind, addressing that issue will need to precede the intermittent fasting plan. The best way to do this is to test both your daily cortisol rhythm and your monthly hormonal cycle with a salivary collection.

Don't diet.

Ok, are you ready for the biggest reason why intermittent fasting DOESN'T work for women? Because we also try to diet at the same time! This is not the concept behind intermittent fasting and will ultimately either lead to bingeing, failure, or health and hormonal issues. During the period of time you are eating, you need to EAT. Eat a lot of really nutrient-dense, calorically-dense foods in that timeframe and do not try to be in a huge calorie deficit. This won't work. I like to think of intermittent fasting as a better, safer, smarter option to restricting calories. But, definitely never do both.

Do focus on fats.

In order to make sure you're not going into too big of a calorie deficit, your diet will need to consist primarily of healthy, nutrient-dense fats. These include fat from properly raised animals, unsweetened coconut and coconut oil, nuts and nut butters, pasture-raised butter or ghee, eggs, avocado and avocado oil, olives and olive oil, and grass-fed dairy products. When these foods become staples, you can rest assured that you will be getting enough nutrients and calories in your day prior to fasting.

Not only that, but switching to a high-fat diet will also ensure your fasting periods are stress-free, safe, and comfortable. With the reduction of carbohydrates and inclusion of a large amount of fat, your blood sugar will become extremely stable. Instead of being a rollercoaster (which is what happens to our blood sugar when we have excess carbohydrates in our diet), it will be more like small waves. When our bodies are on the rollercoaster route, there will be a dip in blood sugar a few hours after your last meal which brings on feelings of hunger. When no glucose is provided by way of a meal, cortisol – our stress hormone – will come to the rescue. So, now you're hungry, you're still fasting for another 5 hours, and your body senses a stressful event. Not good!

However, when you take a high-fat diet approach and become fat-adapted, that dip in blood sugar doesn't happen and the stressor isn't there because your body no longer relies on only glucose for energy. Your body has learned to run on fats – both dietary and stored body fat – instead of just waiting for the next meal. Now, not only are you not having feelings of hunger, but you're eliminating the stressful event! And, as we discussed above, the reason why intermittent fasting can be hard for women is because of the hormonal imbalance that can develop from the stress and cortisol response. Just by eating high-fat and plenty of food, we have eliminated that stressor!

Don't workout intensely.

At least for the first week or two until you know how intermittent will affect you. Once your body becomes adapted to this change, chances are workouts will actually feel better in the fasted state and you will begin to see improvements in your workouts. But, first you need to eliminate all added stressors while your body adapts and gets used to this new energy source (fat). Taking walks in nature or a really great yoga class will be the best way to get movement in during this transition time. After that, begin incorporating short HIIT sessions like jumping rope, sprinting, or heavy lifts in the gym and see how you feel. Remember, the end goal is to keep the stress level in the body at an all time low, thereby keeping your hormones in balance. Working out too intensely while your body is shifting energy sources will likely cause stress.

Don't make fat loss your main goal.

There are many success stories out there of people who have had complete body composition changes just by incorporating intermittent fasting. And it's true. It is a great tool for losing weight, getting leaner, and decreasing body fat. BUT, I don't think any female should do it just for that purpose. This is not the next way to obsess about your body and try to manipulate its size with food.

This is a therapeutic diet with amazing health benefits and should be viewed as such. Find a deeper purpose behind your dietary changes. Do you have brain fog or trouble concentrating? Intermittent fasting is great for brain health. Want to age well and live longer? Intermittent fasting has been shown to prolong lifespan and slow down the aging process. Need to get your blood lipids and cardiovascular markers in check? Intermittent fasting can bring those markers back in range without the use of medication.

Do start slow.

Intermittent fasting isn't something you need to dive into all or nothing for it to be effective. n fact, women may have better luck with easing their way into it. Spend 3-4 weeks becoming fat-adapted with a high fat diet first. Then, add in an intermittent fasting schedule a few days per week. For instance, try doing a 16/8 fast on Monday's and Thursday's and see how that feels. If you enjoy it, add in more days as you feel comfortable.

Don't continue if you feel bad.

This should go without saying, but obviously if you are feeling weak, tired, dizzy, or just don't like it, then don't do it! This is not something that will feel right for everyone, so pay attention, listen to your body, and always do what's right for you.

Do enlist the support of a professional.

As with any advice I give, I always recommend seeking the help of a professional to guide you through the changes you wish to make and support you along the way. This will make it easier to acknowledge what is right for YOU instead of just guessing. If you would like help in determining your individualized plan based on the state of your hormones, contact me for a free 15-minute case review.

So far, we have learned a lot about intermittent fasting and how it affects women and the human body in general. However, there are some mistakes that many newbies make when they dive into intermittent fasting without a plan.

Here is a summary of some of the most common and costly mistakes that you need to avoid:

Continuing to Eat Crap Food

One of the most common complaints people make is that they are following the fasting technique but aren't seeing results. When asked about their nutrition, the answer always reveals the problem. They are still eating processed foods (chips, candy, cake, crackers, etc.) and drinking sweetened beverages (sweet teas and soda). You cannot fast, exercise hard, eat junk food, and still expect that you will lose fat and tone that butt. You must decide to throw away all the unhealthy stuff and go for whole and unprocessed foods. There will be cheat days when you can indulge in something decadent, but don't make that part of your intermittent fasting lifestyle.

Not Keeping Yourself Busy

You cannot spend the day fasting and sitting around doing nothing. Staying idle is the worst thing you can do because you will start thinking about food. Get up and do something to stay active, as long as it keeps you away from food.

You Set Goals Too High

If you are a newbie to intermittent fasting, make sure that you don't start off with only one meal a day. You may think that going in hard from the start will help you torch all that fat, but it doesn't work that way. You cannot go from eating four to six meals a day to surviving on a single meal. You will mess up your hormonal cycles, and the negative effects will outweigh any benefits you gain.

You Fear Going Hungry

It's perfectly normal to feel hungry, but you will not die just because you go for a couple of hours without food. Most people have this irrational and morbid fear of depriving themselves of food, believing that all their muscles will be gobbled up. This fear can tempt you to cheat during your fasting window. Do not be afraid of a bit of hunger.

You Spend Your Days Staring at the Clock

Most newbies will develop an obsession with the clock when fasting. They will count down the hours, minutes, and seconds until they can rush to the kitchen and start bingeing. On the other extreme end are people who are afraid of breaking the "rules," so they make sure that they fast until the last second of the fasting window is over. Intermittent fasting is not that hard or strict. You cannot spend the day worrying and wondering about the timeframes and schedules. If your entire life starts and ends with your next meal, you will drive yourself mad. Just relax and enjoy the ride.

Obsessing Over the Sum of the Parts

Intermittent fasting is like a complex and dynamic system. There are a lot of individual pieces that form a large system. It is useless getting fixated on one small piece and forgetting that there are many more important things to focus on. For example, some people may worry about whether adding a teaspoon of cream to their coffee while fasting will ruin their chances of losing fat. Others wonder whether the 16/8 method is better than the 5:2 Diet. However, there are other bigger concerns that you should be focusing on, for example, your food selection; your training regimen; eating the right portions according to your goals; consuming enough proteins and fats, and so on. The whole is always greater than the sum of the parts. Focus more on spending a portion of your day or week in a fasted state, and the rest of the time feeding normally. Leave the trivialities alone.

Common Myths of Intermittent Fasting

When it comes to losing weight everyone seems to have their own two cents worth of advice to give. Even you have probably offered someone a tip or two about losing weight at one point or another. Today, information is available at the tips of your fingers. You can look up dozens of different weight loss programs on your phone, tablet, computer, in magazines, and books. Most of the time you can't go a day without turning on the television and seeing a commercial for a new "miraculous" supplement, waist shaper, or exercise DVD.

Surveys have shown that more than fifty percent of women in the United States are on a diet at any given moment. So chances are you have already talked to your girlfriends or relatives about fasting and have received a number of different responses. But the fact of the matter is that there are many myths about fasting and intermittent fasting that have become common knowledge that may make you doubt your decision to make this change. In this chapter I am going to debunk the most well- known myths about intermittent fasting, so you understand the full effects of this lifestyle.

Fasting is Basically Starving Yourself

Possibly the greatest myth about fasting is that you
are starving your body of food. Starving obviously
isn't healthy and is attributed to serious eating
disorders. But fasting is not an eating disorder nor is
it starvation. In fact, intermittent fasting helps
individuals develop stable and regular eating habits.
Starvation is when you rob your body of food; you
purposely do not give it any source of food, resulting
in malnourishment and even death. Fasting is when
the participant chooses select times to feed their body
the proper nutrients it needs. Not only are you making
better choices when you fast, but you are also giving
your digestive system a rest. You cannot become
seriously injured or die from fasting, because the
point of intermittent fasting is that you do break the
fast with a delicious meal.

Fasting Will Slow Down Your Metabolism

Your metabolism is the energy used to keep your cells
active and alive, it sustains your life. While it is true
that your metabolic rate effects your weight,
intermittent fasting will not slow it down. Research
has proven time and time again that the quantity of
the food you consume matters, not your eating
pattern. This means that how often you eat or when
you eat does not correlate with your body
composition. What really matters is how much food
you eat in regards to your body composition and
weight. Of course, when it comes to health, quality
matters a great deal as well. Your metabolism is not a
mystical fire that you should try to speed up. It is
something that you should try to optimize. Fasting

will not decrease your metabolism or put your body into starvation mode. Your metabolism will burn however many calories it can, and the only way it will burn more calories for energy is if you also exercise. As long as you eat in a caloric deficit and/ or exercise, you will lose weight.

You Will Gain Back The Weight You Lost After Eating

Another common myth is that fasting is a waste of your time because you will just gain back whatever weight you lose as soon as you stop fasting. The only way you will gain back whatever fat you lost is if you do not adapt fasting as a lifestyle and continuously eat after you stop fasting regularly. Fasting is a long-term (permanent) solution. I understand that your goal with intermittent fasting may be to lose ten or fifteen pounds. But before you began fasting, you knew that you consumed too many calories during the day; that is why you are reading this book. Fasting will reverse your reliance on excess calories. And stopping a fasting lifestyle will in turn reverse your eating habits right back to overeating and consuming excess calories. Intermittent fasting is not a temporary, quick fix solution to losing a few pounds after a few weeks of minimal effort. In that case, you will find yourself right back where you started. The point of fasting then feasting is to plan your meals and make better decisions during your eating period. Weight gain will only occur if you overcompensate during meals by overeating.

Fasting Only Helps You Lose Water Weight

As with many diets, it is a common myth that when you lose weight you are actually losing water weight or muscle glycogen. While this does occur for some people, it is not necessarily true. You absolutely will lose weight in the form of body fat when you fast; it just don't be in the first two weeks of intermittent fasting. As long as you stick to your fasting schedule and plan, you will lose that stubborn belly fat.

Having Less Energy When Fasting

Some people believe that because you are eating less food when you adopt intermittent fasting, you experience a lack of energy. When you first begin fasting, you may experience a slight decrease in energy. But once your mind and body adapt to the change in lifestyle, you will actually have increased energy levels, even when skipping meals. The first week or so is the hardest, as it is with any other lifestyle change. When you are hungry, that is when you will expend the most energy. You can use hunger as motivation to stay strong in your goals and stay active and focused on other important tasks. If you keep yourself distracted throughout your fasting period, intermittent fasting is a much more pleasant experience.

Fat Makes You Fat

Many people choose to adapt much healthier diets when they take on intermittent fasting. One of the most common myths of losing weight through dieting is that eating fat will make you fat. But this is simply not true. Humans cannot live without fats; they are crucial for our survival. But there is a difference between good fats and bad fats. Good fats give us necessary fatty acids and vitamins, energize us, and keep our skin super soft. The combination of bad fats and carbohydrates is what makes people gain weight, not the consumption of fat. There are even studies that have shown a short term high fat, low carb diet will help you lose more weight than other typical dieting methods.

Your Brain Will Stop Functioning Without Carbs

Another myth about dieting and intermittent fasting is that if you do not consume carbohydrates every few hours, your brain will stop working. This belief comes from the theory that your brain can only use glucose to convert to energy. But your body can produce its own glucose through a process called gluconeogenesis. And your body has stored glycogen in the liver that can be used for energy. Lastly, long-term fasting or low carb diets will force your body to produce ketone bodies, which will also energize your brain. The fact of the matter is that our bodies are more than capable of surviving without a constant supply of carbohydrates. If this was not the case, humans would have been extinct long ago.

You Need Supplements To Make Up for Lack of Food

There are dozens of different supplements that "experts" claim your body needs during a fasting period. But you don't need green tea pills or raspberry ketones to lose weight and stay motivated during your fast. All your body needs is water.

Fasting and Training Are a Bad Combination

While some aerobic activities, such as running, may have a slight negative impact on performance, anaerobic performance, like lifting weights is not as effected by intermittent fasting. Although carbohydrates boost your energy while exercising, a key factor to a good workout is staying hydrated. The most common type of athlete that participates in intermittent fasting is a weight trainer or lifter. And luckily for athletes who are focused on changing their body composition, fasting allows your body to lose fat while still gaining muscle: as long as you feast with the right kinds of food.

When Fasting Is Not For Everyone ...

As you now know, fasting can effect women differently than men; which means that there are limitations to who can or should fast and who cannot. There are also a number of other factors that come into play when deciding if you should fast, like stress and eating disorders.

You should not try intermittent fasting if:

•   You are pregnant - This is because pregnant women have a higher demand for more energy and nutrients that come from what they eat and drink. But really, some women should not even try experimenting with intermittent fasting at all. If you do not feast or fast properly, you risk become infertile or early onset menopause: even if you are in your twenties.

•	You having a history of any kind of eating disorder – Individuals who have suffered from an eating disorder are more likely to develop another eating disorder at some point in their lives. Fasting and feasting could lead patients with unhealthy eating patterns to develop additional problems.

•	You are chronically stressed or do not handle physical or mental stress well – people who experience constant chronic stress should not limit their diet or meals because they may actually need more nourishment.

•	You have insomnia or unusual sleeping habits – Just like individuals with chronic stress, if you have trouble sleeping, then you need to be nurturing your body not adding more stress.

•	If you are new to exercising and dieting and this is the first time you are trying a new lifestyle.

Now that you fully understand the science behind fasting, as well as the many benefits and myths behind the method, you are now prepared to read all about the different types of intermittent fasting plans. Everyone has their own needs when it comes to incorporating a new lifestyle; Jill may work a full time job and have a family to take care of, while Katie is a full time student who works out five days a week. Whatever your needs are, there is a way to adopt intermittent fasting without it disrupting your everyday life.

Conclusion

If you want to stick to intermittent fasting for life, then you must not view it as a diet but as a life style. This will require you to reevaluate your eating choices even before beginning the fast so that when you begin, you are sure that you won't be going back. For example, if you use regular vegetable oil then it is time to replace it with healthy oils such as coconut oil and olive oil. If you tend to eat processed carbs then it is time to replace them with healthy whole unprocessed carbs- e.g. zucchini noodles in place of pasta.

The idea here is to embrace the diet and the fact that your body will be a full on fat burning means that new carbs won't be required for body fuel. It will typically take a few weeks for this to happen but once it does, cravings for unhealthy carbs will be out of the picture and incorporating this diet into your life will be as easy as ABC.

If you are going to live the ultimate intermittent fasting lifestyle then:

The best way to include Intermittent Fasting into your life style is by delaying your breakfast slowly by slowly- delay by an hour then another hour the next day and so on. Take an hour to shower, an hour to do your chores, an hour to get to work- just take an hour from any activity that you engage in the morning that you see best fit until you get to a time that you can live with.

Do not use fasting as an excuse to eat junk- calories are different. 100 calories of broccoli are not the same as 100 calories of a snicker bar. When you find yourself cheating then get real with yourself. Keep the carbs for before work outs and fill yourself up with meats and veggies.

Stick to the method that you are most comfortable with- as discussed, there are a number of ways to do intermittent fasting. Play around with all of them and get what suits you best. Make sure you actually try out all methods- you might be surprised which will be easiest to follow. In order to make something part of your lifestyle, you need to be fully comfortable with it. Intermittent fasting is no different.